YOUR KNOWLEDGE HAS VALUE

- We will publish your bachelor's and master's thesis, essays and papers

- Your own eBook and book - sold worldwide in all relevant shops

- Earn money with each sale

Upload your text at www.GRIN.com
and publish for free

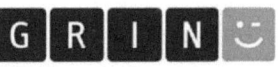

Bibliographic information published by the German National Library:

The German National Library lists this publication in the National Bibliography; detailed bibliographic data are available on the Internet at http://dnb.dnb.de .

Imprint:

Copyright © 2015 GRIN Verlag, Open Publishing GmbH
Print and binding: Books on Demand GmbH, Norderstedt Germany
ISBN: 9783668470910

This book at GRIN:

http://www.grin.com/en/e-book/368322/knowledge-attitude-and-practise-of-front-line-health-professionals-towards

Sharew Niguse

Knowledge, Attitude and Practise of Front Line Health Professionals towards MDR-TB Prevention and its Associated Factors with the Practice in Addis Abeba

GRIN Publishing

GRIN - Your knowledge has value

Since its foundation in 1998, GRIN has specialized in publishing academic texts by students, college teachers and other academics as e-book and printed book. The website www.grin.com is an ideal platform for presenting term papers, final papers, scientific essays, dissertations and specialist books.

Visit us on the internet:

http://www.grin.com/

http://www.facebook.com/grincom

http://www.twitter.com/grin_com

DEBREMARKOS UNIVERSITY AND GAMBY COLLEGE OF MEDICAL SCIENCE JOINT MPH PROGRAM

KNOWLEDGE, ATTITUDE AND PRACTICE OF FRONT LINE HEALTH PROFESSIONALS TOWARDS MDR TB PREVENTION AND ITS ASSOCIATED FACTORS WITH THE PRACTICE IN ADDIS ABABA

NAME OF AUTHOR: SHAREW NIGUSE

A THESIS SUBMITTED TO THE PUBLIC HEALTH DEPARTMENT, DEBRE MARKOS UNIVERSITY IN PARTIAL FULFILLMENT OF THE REQUIREMENTS FOR THE DEGREE OF MASTTER OF PUBLIC HEALTH

August, 2015

Addis Ababa, Ethiopia

Acknowledgement

My deepest acknowledgment for this thesis work development given to my advisors, Moges Wubie and CheruTesemafor their valuable supports during the development of this proposal. Starting from the beginning of proposal development their contribution to shape the scope of this study was highly appreciated.

My thanks alsowill go toZewdieAdraw for his honest, heartfelt and enthusiast support starting from topic selection to write up with diverse aspect of support for the fruitful work of this paper.

This thesis work come to its end with the help of my friends Melaku Anjelo and Bahailu Fantahun in coordinating the data collection process; taking this paceI would like to say thank you so much for their genuine support.

Lastly I would like to acknowledge Debremarkos University and GAMBY college of Medical Science Joint MPH program for giving me such a chance and advising me in doing this thesis work.

Contents

List of Tables

List of Figures

Acronyms

BCG-	BacilleCalmette-Guérin
CDC-	center for disease control
DOT-	Direct Observed Treatment
OPD-	outpatient department
HIV-	Human immune deficiency virus
IGRAs-	inferior gamma release assays
KAP –	knowledge attitude and practice
LED-	light emitting diodes
LPA-	line probe assay
LTBI -	latent tuberculosis infection
MDR TB-	multi drug resistance tuberculosis
TB-	tuberculosis
WHO-	world health organization
XDR TB-	extensive drug resistance tuberculosis

ABSTRACT

INTRODUCTION: Tuberculosis is an infection caused by Mycobacterium tuberculosis and most of the time affects lung (pulmonary tuberclosis). When it is not treated effectively it will develop resistance to medication and it will results in drug resistance tuberculosis. Globally, 3.5% of new and 20.5% of previously treated tuberclosis cases was estimated to have had Multi-Drug Resistance Tuberculosis in 2013. One of the factors of an increase for Multi drug resistance tuberculosis is the health professionals' Knowledge, attitude and practice towards MDR TB prevention. Hence, this study will have contributed an input for further studies.

OBJECTIVE: to assessment of the knowledge, attitude and practice of frontline health worker towards MDR TB prevention and its associated factors in Addis Ababa by the year 2015.

METHODS: A cross sectional study design was used. This study was conducted in Addis Ababa from March18- April 30/2015. Three hundred twelve health professionals from 18 health centers in Addis Ababa of all sub cities were included in the study. Semi-structured self-administered questionnaire used to collect dataand each questionnaire collected anonymously. Data entry and analysis was done using SPSS 20. The output here under presented using text, graph and table. Binary logistic and multiple logisticregressions werecomputed.

RESULT: a total of 312 people participated in this study and 59.9% of them were female. The knowledge score of frontline health professionals have a value of 59.6%. Around 70.8% of frontline health professionals have favorable attitude for the practice of MDR TB prevention. 58.65% of health professionals have good practice. The knowledge of health professionals were significantly associated with the practice of frontline health professionals towards MDR TB prevention with AOR00:3.807[2.095, 6.919].About 183(58.65%) of frontline health professionals have good practice with a mean score of 49.2.

CONCLUSION: with a poor knowledge score, frontline health professional practice towards MDR TB prevention was strongly associated with their knowledge hence, Addis Ababa health Bureau and it partners should work to improve the knowledge of health professionals towards MDR TB prevention.

Key words: frontline health professionals, Knowledge, attitude, practice, Addis Ababa Ethiopia.

6

1. INTRODUCTION

1.1 BACKGROUND

Tuberculosis (TB) is an infection caused by mycobacterium tuberculosis. No matter it is curable disease it kills close to 2 million people around the world each year. Its impact is greatest on adults in their most productive working years (ages 15-54). Two billion people are infected with TB worldwide, nearly one-third of the global population. Of nine million new tuberculosis cases each year, nearly half a million are multidrug-resistant tuberculosis (MDR-TB). China and India account for 50 percent of MDR-TB cases worldwide. Multidrug-resistant tuberculosis (MDR-TB) is a major global public health threat resulting from interrupted or incomplete treatment of TB. MDR-TB does not respond to standard TB drugs, and treatment relies on a handful of antibiotics. The treatment for MDR-TB is long and complex, often resulting in poor patient compliance and development of further drug resistance (1).

Resistance to anti-TB drugs can occur when the drugs are misused or mismanaged. Examples include when patients do not complete their full course of treatment; when health-care providers prescribe the wrong treatment, the wrong dose, or length of time for taking the drugs; when the supply of drugs is not always available; or when the drugs are of poor quality. Drug-resistant TB (MDR or XDR) is more common in people who do not take their TB medicine regularly, do not take all of their TB medicines as prescribed by their doctor, develop TB disease again after having taken TB medicine in the past, come from areas of the world where drug-resistant TB is common and have spent time with someone known to have drug-resistant TB disease (2).

Some TB control programs have shown that cure is possible for an estimated 30% to 50% of affected people with XDR TB. Successful outcomes depend greatly on the extent of the drug resistance, the severity of the disease, whether the patient's immune system is weakened, and adherence to treatment (3).

TB can be diagnosed in different way, using molecular, bacteriological, pictographically and radiological diagnostic method. Most commonly used method of TB diagnosis is bacteriological method of diagnosis. Sputum microscopy is one of the most applicable methods of diagnosis in Ethiopia. It is most efficient and applicable method to identify infectious TB cases in peripheral laboratories. It is used for diagnosis, monitoring and

7

defining cure. Three sputum specimens must be collected and examined in two consecutive days. Light emitting diode (LED) microscopy is a newly introduced diagnostic tool to complement the conventional microscopy. It is recommended for centers with high case load as it saves time and improves sensitivity (4).

The knowledge, attitude and practice of health professionals is one of the decisive factor for preventing and control of MDR TB since they are the one who is responsible in treating and counseling patients for successful adherence of treatment. But there is a situation where we can find health professionals with a serious knowledge gap, unfavorable attitude and poor practice to prevent MDR TB. A study conducted in Lima, Peru indicated that most of the health professionals had very good knowledge on means of transmission and the contagious nature of TB however, only 21.9% of the surveyed professionals including less than half of doctors and nurses recognized that not all patients with TB develops symptoms. In addition to this only 30.1% of the surveyed professionals know that the correct way of diagnosing TB is through sputum. Furthermore, less than half of the respondents recognized that drug resistant TB or its spread were the result of inadequate or incomplete treatment. Understanding the problem is one part of the solution for MDR TB prevention; hence having continues research work is very important to set the right solution (5).

1.2 STATEMENT OF THE PROBLEM

TB is one of the highest killer diseases in this world, 6 million people will die each year with malaria, HIV and TB; out of this nearly 2 million deaths is dues to TB. Even though TB is curable disease 5000 people is dying due to TB every day. What makes the situation worse is the highest share of the disease share will fall in the developing country (98% of death due to TB is among developing country affecting younger age in their most productive age) (6).

Frontline health professionals are at risk of developing TB and MDR TB infections. A retrospective cohort study done in South Africa, KwaZulu-Natal show that from a total of 1,313 (92%) medical chart reviewed 112(9%) cases were identified. Among total patient of health worker with TB 14(13%) of them had MDR TB, 36 (32%) were cured, 13(12%) of them were died. Health worker that works in TB ward had increased rate of infection as compared to other wards (7).

There is a gap on the knowledge, attitude and practice of health worker towards MDR TB prevention. a study conducted in Maluti Adventist hospital, South Africa showed even though most of the respondents (89.2%) of them had good knowledge on the transmission diagnosis and prevention of TB, only (22%) of them know the appropriate sputum collection. More than one third (36.4%) of the respondents reported poor practice of the infection control(8).

Effective follow up and tracing of TB patient is significant for proper management of TB and prevention of the development of MDR TB. However, the study conducted on the knowledge, practice and challenge of tracing TB patient for an improved adherence to treatment, in South Africa indicated 50-59.3% of the tracer group were able to identify four components of DOT encounters. This matter the management of TB patients whether to give health education our counseling on treatment Adherence in the long run its contribution to an increase in the burden of MDR TB is very high(9).

Working with the national treatment guideline on treatment of TB is one of the recommended good practices to prevent MDR TB, nevertheless, a study conducted in Addis Ababa showed that health care providers have been using National Treatment Guideline while diagnosing patients only for 60.9% of female patients and 56.4% of male patients. Despite the fact that there were correct prescriptions of TB pills for 90.2% of female patients and 91.8% of male patients, both under and over prescription were occurred. Surprisingly only 2.6% of smear negative TB patients had been diagnosed correctly. This indicates that there is a serious gap on the knowledge and practice of health professionals on prevention of MDR TB (10).

Ethiopia is one of the country where there is a very high magnitude of TB infections available .An estimate TB burden by WHO indicates that only 22 country contribute 80% of TB burden and Ethiopia rank 8th following India, China, Indonesia, Nigeria, Bangladesh, Pakistan and south Africa (11).

Though there is an effort to reduce and curve the transmission rate of TB in Ethiopia still a lot has to be done to reach the intended goal. In a country like Ethiopia where the prevalence of TB and HIV co-infection is very high there should be continues research program need to be in place and the country developed TB road map operational research program. According to this research program one of the priority research areas is MDR TB (12).

In a country like Ethiopia the problem of TB will be very high as compared to developed country where the life style of people is highly inevitable for high transmission of TB. In

Ethiopian people usually share single room for a number of people and if one of them got TB the likely hood of TB transmission in the house is very high(13).

Therefore, conducting this study to assess the knowledge attitude and practice of front line health professionals on MDR TB prevention is significant and will contribute an input to plan resource for prevention of MDR TB in Addis Ababa.

1.3 LITRATURE REVIEW

Globally, 3.5% of new and 20.5% of previously treated TB cases were estimated to have had MDR-TB in 2013. This translates into an estimated 480 000 people having developed MDR-TB in 2013.On average, an estimated 9.0% of patients with MDRTB had extensively drug resistant TB (XDR-TB).If all notified TB patients (6.1 million, new and previously treated) had been tested for drug resistance in 2013, an estimated 300 000 cases of MDR-TB would have been detected, more than half of these in three countries alone: India, China and the Russian Federation (14).

Tuberculosis is one and the most serious disease that impose highest burden on the economic condition of the country. Studies done in china where the prevalence of TB is very high indicates that the average assets for TB case was 21812 Yuan which is significantly less than the control household asset of 24489, one third of the new case income quintile (0-16699) compared to one fifth of the control (15).

Another study from India tells us the same fact that TB has an enormous socio economic impact on the family and the country at last. TB patient incurs out of pocket money of 5986 Rs to 13,000 crores a year for the country. 11% of the children dropped out of school due to the illness of their parent and 20% of children will be forced to enroll to employment to support the family life (16).

Health professional knowledge and attitude is the most fundamental in addressing and changing the attitude of the community on TB prevention and control whenever the knowledge of health professional is very poor the impact on the community that come to health service delivery area will be impacted. Health professionals starting their undergraduate study the level of knowledge will have an impact when they started work in the real life situation as the study indicates from Italy 2,220 from different 15 universities were included in the study and out of this only 60% of them were able to answer question about clinical and vaccine detail of TB (17).

In majority of settings people prefer to consult health professionals about their health problem. studies from Tajikistan Of the 509 migrants asked what are the top three sources to effectively reach people with information on TB,78% indicated the television, 61% the health workers, and 36% the radio (18).

Study from Peru, Lima indicates that only 67% of the health professionals scored relatively highest, from the total 15 knowledge questions they answered 10, $\pm$ 1.7 89.4% of the study participants agreed that there is difficulty of convincing the patients to continue taking their medication after they fell well from their pain (19)

The study conducted in South Africa about knowledge, attitude and practice of preventing multidrug-resistance tuberculosis at BostabeloHospital Maseru, Lesotho shows only 47.3% of the health professionals have good knowledge about MDR TB even though there is difference between health professionals, 83.3% among doctors and 28.6% among counsellors. As indicated by the study though the attitude was not influenced by good knowledge (85% of them have negative attitude) good knowledge of the health professional was highly associated with goodpractice mask use, p-value =0.01 and referring TB treatment guideline, p-value= 0.03 (20).

The attitude of health professional also one of the factor for improper treatment follow up and defaulters which potentially resulted in increasing the burden of TB in any country where the attitude of the health professional is not good. A study from South Africa indicates one of the factors for increase rate of defaulter in TB treatment is the attitude of the health professionals. The study includes a total of 3165 patients from 8 different provinces where 1164 (232 cases and 932 controls) were traceable and interviewed about the risk factors for defaulting and one of the significant risk factor for both control and case were poor attitude among health care workers (new: AOR 2.1,95%CI and 1.1 for re-treatment) (21).

Another study conducted in Nigeria, Plateau state on the knowledge and attitude of health professionals towards MDR TB showed only 43.4% of them know what kind of action they have to take when the patient miss their treatment in the intensive phase and 71.1% of them lack knowledge on the duration of the treatment with unfriendly attitude towards the patients. Within the same country in the southern part of Nigeria another study was conducted to assess the level of knowledge of health professionals towards MDR TB and more than one third(38.5%) of them had poor knowledge (22, 23).

11

A study done in Addis Ababa about the determinates of MDR TB in Addis Ababa show that one of the factor for increase burden of MDR TB is due to less follow up of patient by health professionals. According to this study 29% of the cases perceived that the care from health professional was poor. And one of the reasons for MDR TB is follow up during the first line treatment of TB. Among MDR TB patients only 51% of them observed by health professionals as compared to 94.8% of the control were followed by health professional according to the strict DOT guideline of the country (24).

In Ethiopia a total of 503 MDR TB patient was initiated the treatment out of these 444 were from Addis Ababa and 59 were from Gondar. Almost all were on good follow up of their treatment that is 100% adherence to treatment. The same year 243 out patients and 55 in patients in Addis Ababa and 38 out patients and 12 in patients in Gondar 9 patients presumed to have extremely drug resistance TB. 9.8% of the patient died and 1.2% interrupted the treatment (25).

1.4 SIGNIFICANCE OF THE STUDY

Conducting this study in Addis Ababa have great input to prevent MDR TB, because it can give a clue on the status of the knowledge, attitude and practice of health professionals that work in Addis Ababa health facilities

Mainly this study have primary importance for Addis Ababa city administration health bureau for planning of resources to give an appropriate training for those health professionals that work under health centers in all Addis Ababa to prevent TB infection.

In addition, this study has an importance to the study participants themselves, the finding of this study recommended the necessary modalities that each health professionals will have information about TB based on the gap obtained here in the study.

Another benefits of this study will be for the community, whenever the knowledge, attitude and practice of health professionals get improved the access to information about TB, the access to good counseling about TB and related problem will be improved and the sum effect will result in reducing the burden of TB and MDR TB will reduce in the country and the economic loss as a result of this health problem will be managed.

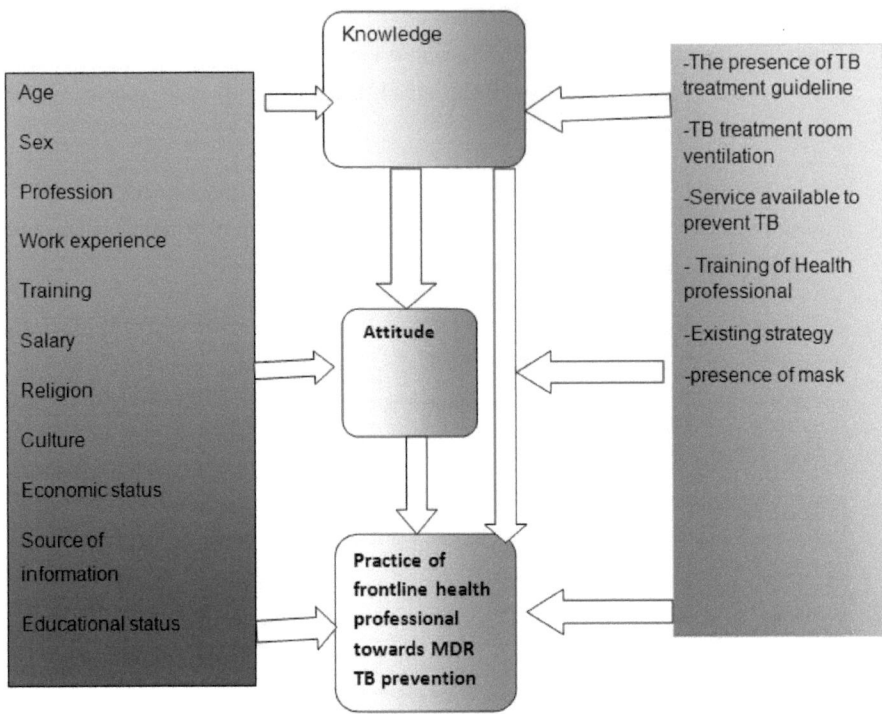

Figure 1 conceptual framework

2. OBJECTIVE

2.1 General objective

To assess the knowledge attitude and practice of frontline health workers towards MDR TB and factors associated with the practice of MDR TB prevention in Addis Ababa by the year 2015.

2.2 Specific objectives

1. To determine the level of knowledge of frontline health professionals towards MDR TB.
2. To determine the level of attitude of frontline health professionals towards MDR TB
3. To determine the level of frontline health professional practice towards MDR TB prevention
4. To identify factors associated with the practice of MDR TB prevention by frontline health professionals.

3. METHODS

3.1 Study design

A cross sectional study design was used to conduct this study.

3.2 Study area/Study Period

The study was conducted in Addis Ababa,the capital city of Ethiopia since the early 1900s. According to the Central Statistics Agency the city had 3,104,000 population as of july 2013. Addis Ababa has 10 sub city and 116 Woredas.

Addis Ababa has 41 hospital out of this 10 of them are public while the rest 31 of them owned by private investors and nonprofit organizations. Currently Addis Ababa has 86 health centers, 80 of them fully functioning while the rest graduated and not yet started to give service to the public.

3.3 Population

3.3.1 Source population

The source population for this study was frontline health professionals that work under health centers in Addis Ababa, working under OPD, TB clinics and laboratory. According to the human resource data of Addis Ababa health bureau the total frontline health professional that work under those departments estimated to be 1720.

3.3.2 Study population

The study population was those frontline health workers working under OPD, TB clinics and laboratory from the selected health centers.

3.4 Sample size & sampling procedures

The sample size was calculated based on single population proportion formula having the following assumptions: Using $n = \frac{Z^2\ PxQ}{W2}$

$n = \frac{(1.96^2)(0.5*0.5)}{(0.05)2} \cong 384$

Where, Z^2 is a standard score for 95% confidence interval?

P is 50% of the proportion

Q is the probability of losing the proportion

W=margin of error between sample and the population.

Since we don't have the prevalence of health professionals' knowledge attitude and practice in Addis Ababa 50% used in order to obtain maximum sample size for each dependent variable.

Since the study population was small the sample size was adjusted and gave ≅315. Considering 10% nonresponsive rate the total population that will be included in the study will be **347**.Based on the information collected from Addis Ababa Health office the total number of health professionals that work under OPD, Laboratory and TB clinics on average was 20 and a total sample size taken divided by this number gives ≅18 and study participants included from 18 health centers. Each health centers included in the study identified like this: a total number of health centers that were fully functioning i.e.80/18=4.4, hence every 5 health centers included in the study using the arranged list obtained from Addis Ababa health bureau.

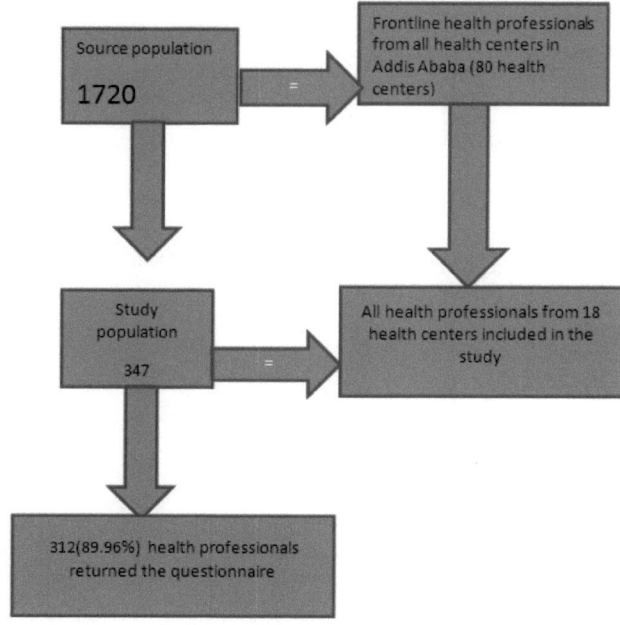

Figure 2 Summary of sampling procedure

3.5 Inclusion and exclusion criteria

3.5.1 Inclusion criteria

Those health professional works under OPD, TB clinics and Laboratory permanently were included in the study.

3.5.2 Exclusion criteria

Health professionals who are away from their job during the data collection period due to different reason like disciplinary suspension, serious illness and other social circumstance will not be included due to feasibility of the study.

3.6 Variable

3.6.1 Dependent variables

* Practice of front line health professionals towards MDR TB prevention

3.6.2 Independent variables

* Age
* Sex
* Profession
* Work experience
* Training
* Salary
* Religion
* Economic status
* Source of information
* Educational status
* Knowledge
* Attitude

3.7 Operational definitions

Front line health worker (FHW) - are those health professionals who work under health center from the selected health centers OPD,TB clinics and Laboratory department since health center is the primary treatment unit in Addis Ababa.

Good knowledge- whose health professionals that answered ≥80% of the given questionnaire correctly from the given question.

Insufficient knowledge- those health professionals answered less than <80% of the question correctly.

Favorable attitude- question given score from 1-5 from strongly negative to strongly positive for each question and hence those who scored above 3 was considered as having favorable attitude in preventing MDR TB

Unfavorable attitude- those who scored less than or equal to 3 was regarded as unfavorable attitude to prevent MDR TB

Good practice-frontline health professionals that scored greater than or equal to mean valueout of 10 practice question regarded as having good practice.

Poor practice- frontline health professionals who scored less than the mean valuefrom a total of 10 practice question regarded as having poor practice.

3.8 Data collection tool and procedure

Data collectors which have at least one year experience in the field of data collection were recruited to facilitate this self-administered questionnaire. The knowledge of front line health professionals were assessed using 12 questions with multiple choices. The attitude of frontline health professionals were assessed using 12 questions and each questionnaire were given scale (Likert scale). The practice of health professionals were assessed using a total of 10 questions while 3 of them were the main focus and the rest were supportive to those 3 questions. The data was collected by self-administered method. Once after the questionnaire filled by each health professional it was dropped in the pre-designed box with a sealed envelope to collect the information anonymously.

3.9 Data quality management

Five health centers from five different sub-cities which are not selected for the study was chosen and pretest conducted. The pre-test was included 5% (18) of the study population and intended to check whether the tools enable to collect the intended information without any ambiguity. Each respondent was oriented how to fill the data independently. Respondents were told to make sure that there is no missing information before they seal the envelope through rechecking mechanism. Based on the sample calculated the number of

19

health centers needed was considered first and in order to avoid selection bias list of health centers used as frame. Systematic sampling method used to select those sampled health centers and all of health professionals from the selected health centers included in the study. In order to avoid information and social desirability bias each questionnaire was kept inside an envelope and given to the respondents. Once after the respondents completed filling the questionnaire they enclosed it inside an envelope sealing it and drooped inside the box specifically designed in the compound for this purpose. While the respondents fill this questionnaire they had been informed that they will not write any labeling that indicate their personal information.

3.9.1 Data Processing and Analysis

The data entry and analysis was done using SPSS20.The output of data presented here using graphs, cross table and charts. Bi-variate and multi-variateanalysiswas computed to see the association between the practice of health professionals and other factors. P- Value of 0.25 was taken as cut of point to continue doing multivariate analysis andP-value =0.05 was taken as cut off point for the significant of factors with the dependant variables.

3.10 Ethical considerations

The letter of acceptance of this proposal was written from the university of Debremarkos and GAMBY College of Medical Science research ethical review committee. After the letter of acceptance received from the research ethical review committee this thesis proposal and letter of acceptance was submitted to Addis Ababa health bureau for further review and permission to run the study within the city administration. Once after the proposal and letter submitted to Addis Ababa health bureau; the research ethical committee of the Addis Ababa health bureau approved it. Following letter written from Addis Ababa health bureau each sub-city wrote another letter for respective health centers. Then proper orientation given to health center heads and study participants how they can fill the questionnaire and all issue of confidentiality. As part of the orientation the study participants was clearly told that all the information collected with this study will not be shared and individual has the right to participate and will not be forced to be part of the study with clear explanation that both participating and not in this study will not have direct benefit and disadvantage. Each participant of the study got an information on as this study is for academic purpose the outcome of the study will benefit both parts equally; this information clearly transferred to all participants and they informed that once after they fill each questionnaire they will drop in to a box designed under sealed envelope to collect the information within the compound.

4. RESULTS

4.1 Socio demographic characteristics of the respondents

This study included a total of 347 participants and out of this 312 (89.91%) of them had returned the questionnaire while the remaining 35 professionals didn't returned due to different reasons like the absence of the respondents at the time of collection and they didn't put in the collection boxes prepared for this study purpose.

In this study from a total of 312 individuals included in the study, 186(59.6%) of them were female. Regarding the age of the study respondents, this study included participants with age range between 20 and 50 with a mean age of 28. When we see the religion composition of the study participants, the highest percentage is orthodox Christianity 223(71.47%). The average income of the study participants in this study was 2900 with a maximum of 8000 birr and minimum of 1233. Regarding to educational status of the study participants the highest percentage was degree holder followed by diploma. Regarding the training attended about TB/MDR TB in the past one year only 82(26.28%) of the participants got training. Most of the study participants use book as their source of information about TB followed by media 184(58.97%) and 58(18.59%) respectively(table 1).